So Sweet You Are
You Crazy Beauty,
And So Dear
To Them All!

- Mihai Eminescu, *"Atit de Dulce"*

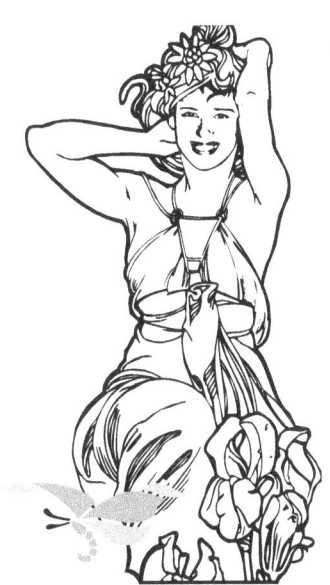

For over ninety years four generations of my family have been enjoying the benefits of these recipes. Why don't you, too?

Transform your makeup table in a home beauty salon and treat your skin with the secret powers of fruits. Learn how to make your own favorite face masks and cleansers by using only fresh fruits, vitamins and natural oils.

All these tips, and many more now-revealed beauty secrets, will remind you how beautiful and sexy you are.

Stay that way!

Stephanie

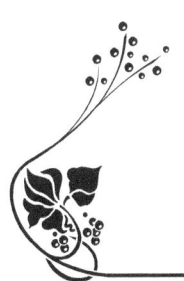

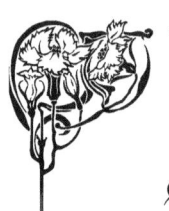

Stephanie's Home Beauty Salon

MAKE YOUR OWN FACE MASKS
FROM FRUITS, VITAMINS AND NATURAL OILS

///

Beauty recipes written by
Stephanie Darie

First Edition
Published in Canada, October 1996
ISBN 0-96812-460-7

Second Edition
Published in the United States, May 2008
ISBN 1438225059 / EAN-13 9781438225050

///

Some of this book's artwork was adapted from
Ted Menten's book of copyright-free resources
"Art Nouveau Small Frames and Borders".
General Publishing Company
Toronto, 1987

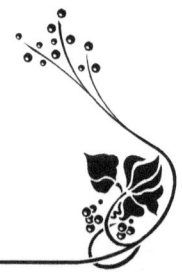

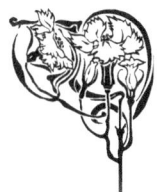

Not A Medical Reference

THIS COLLECTION OF RECIPES IS NOT A MEDICAL REFERENCE!

If you believe in the powerful relationship between nature, health and beauty, then this is the book for you! This is a book about beauty and self-esteem. This is not, however, a medical reference.

Since first published in 1996, the recipes in this book have been used successfully by hundreds of women with all skin types who, while maintaining healthy and beautiful-looking skin complexions, also managed to build priceless self-esteems. The author herself, has been using these recipes regularly for over twenty years.

Throughout the content of this collection, we made notes as to the appropriate use of each recipe and, in an effort to provide you with some contextual terminology, at the end of the book we included a small glossary of basic terms. However, for full professional advice and complete information regarding different definitions of skin types, problems or treatments that you may be searching for, you should consult a dermatologist. Please note that this collection of skin creams does not contain information on the treatment of any specific skin problems including acne, rosacea or other related medical conditions.

If you have serious skin problems, or are allergic to (certain) fruits, you are advised not to use this collection of recipes as a potential remedy. If that is your case, we strongly recommend that you see your dermatologist for professional advice on skin treatments.

Do not use these recipes as substitutes to your physician's advice. Should you, however, decide to use these recipes for beauty purposes, we recommend that you use only natural fresh fruits as opposed to scented or flavored simulates that may appear to replace the genuine. Still, as each of us is unique, results may vary. Not all recipes may give the same described result(s) for everyone. Not all recipes my apply to you.

The final decision as to whether to use these recipes or not, lies with you. You understand that by purchasing this book, and by making use of the information contained in this collection of skin cream recipes, you agree to waive your right to hold liable the author of these recipes and the publisher of this book, as to any kind of direct or consequential health, or otherwise, damages that may occur from your decision to use these recipes.

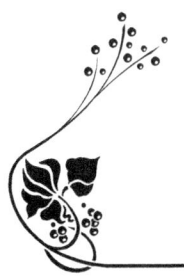

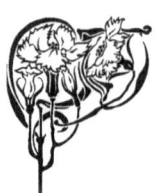

Index of Recipes *By Skin Types*

Normal Skin Complexion

Dry Skin Complexion

Oily Skin Complexion

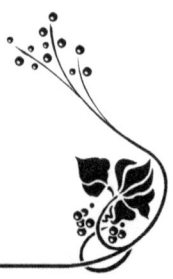

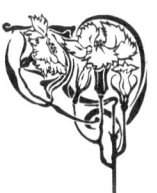

Table of Contents and Recipes

By Fruits in Alphabetical Order

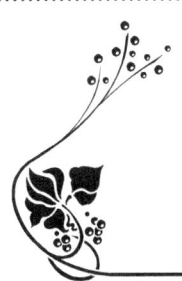

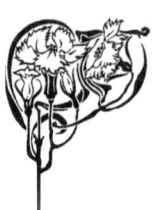

Apple - Malus Communis

Health and Beauty Benefits

As a rich source of flavonoid and polyphenols, apple has excellent soothing properties for dry skin. Apple cider vinegar has exfoliating properties (thus, a good remedy for dandruff removal); when mixed with honey apple cider becomes a very powerful natural energizer and healer.

Natural Properties

Apple contains water, sugar, pectin, malic, tartaric and citric acids and is a rich source of flavonoid and polyphenols which are powerful antioxidants. The pectin in apple helps remove toxic substances that accumulate in skin's surface over time.

Vitamins: A, B, and C
Minerals: Calcium, Copper, Iodine, Iron, Magnesium, Manganese and Phosphorus.

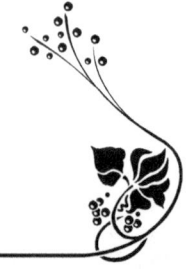

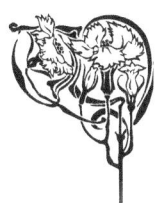

Apple as Skin Cleanser
Dry Skin Complexion

What you need

1 red apple

What to do

Take one big, red apple and, without peeling it, put it in a squeezer, press and collect its delicious juice. Warm up the juice to a moderate temperature and then let it sit for about ten minutes in order to settle. Now it's a good time to wash your face with warm water and soap, then dry it with a paper towel in order to prevent any germs from penetrating your skin. Now, that the pores of your skin are open, the only thing you want it to absorb is the apple juice you've just have prepared.

Pour the warm apple juice in your favorite cosmetic bowl and, using a cotton pad, apply it thoroughly to your face. Relax for about 15 minutes while the juice is being absorbed. After that, wash your face with warm water and, once again, dry it off with a paper towel. Soon you will notice a very fresh and relaxed feel of your skin. Repeat this process as often as you like.

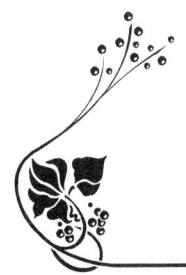

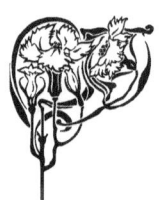

Apple - Malus Communis

Health and Beauty Benefits

For centuries, apple has been used both as a source of food and a powerful natural remedy and is probably the best nutrition element that you will ever treat your skin with. Being very alkaline in composition, apple cider vinegar is beneficial in balancing the body's pH levels.

Apple soothes the skin, relaxes face muscles and delays the formation of wrinkles. Apple can also be used on sunburned areas.

Natural Properties

Vitamins: A, B, and C
Minerals: Calcium, Copper, Iodine, Iron, Magnesium, Manganese and Phosphorus.

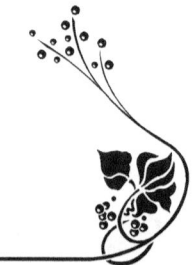

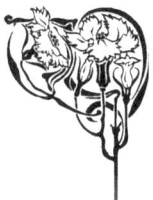

Apple and Milk as Skin Nutrients

Dry Skin Complexion

What you need

> 1 apple
> 250 grams of 2% milk
> 500 grams of mineral water

What to do

Slice one fresh apple and boil it in milk at moderate heat for five minutes. Stir often while boiling. When it is done, pull the apple slices out of the milk and crush them in a blender for 30 seconds while they are still warm.

Apply this cleansing milk on your face with a cosmetic sponge. Leave on the face for fifteen minutes and then remove it with mineral water.

Soon you will feel an unmatched, long-lasting, refreshing feel of your skin.

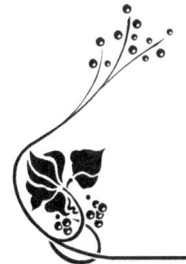

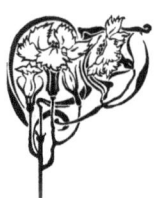

Apricot - Armeniaca Vulgaris

Health and Beauty Benefits

Apricot is also an effective skin lubricant with excellent moisturizing and softening effects. Use this practice in order to regain your skin's vitality through a daily, ten minutes massage.

This process will also rebalance your skin's supply of water. Just as in the application of the apricot mask, your face will benefit here from the same vitamins and minerals, only at a slightly higher concentration this time.

Enjoy your fresh, smooth sensation.

Natural Properties

Vitamins: A, B, C, and E
Minerals: Brume, Chrome, Iron, Magnesium, Potassium and Sulfur.

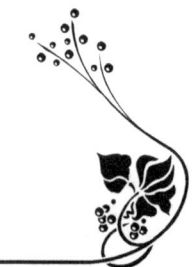

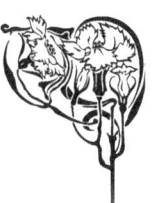

Apricot Cream for Face & Body Massage *Dry Skin Complexion*

What you need

    1 fresh apricot

What to do

Wash your face with warm water. While still moist, apply two halves of a fresh apricot and gently massage the skin for about ten minutes. Apricot has a high content of vitamin E which, during massaging, is rapidly absorbed by your skin.

When finished, wash your face gently with a cosmetic sponge soaked in warm chamomile infusion. Repeat once a day for one week, then every other day for the second week. Only a repeated process of a moisturizing solution will rebalance your skin's supply of water.

This is something you can use this for both your face and throughout your body.

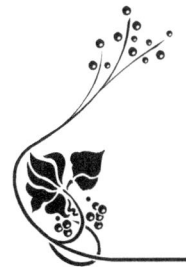

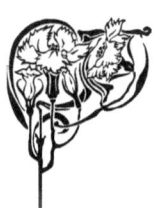

Apricot - Armeniaca Vulgaris

Health and Beauty Benefits

As I mentioned in the previous recipe, among other health and beauty benefits, apricot is an effective skin lubricant with excellent moisturizing and softening effects.

However, when mixed with bee honey and sour cream, apricot has excellent anti-wrinkle properties and is a wonderful face nerve relaxant.

This recipe you will want to prepare according to your complexion, but before that, you will also need to prepare a small bowl of chamomile extract. See pages 22 and 23.

Natural Properties

Vitamins: A, B, C, and E
Minerals: Brume, Chrome, Iron, Magnesium, Potassium and Sulfur.

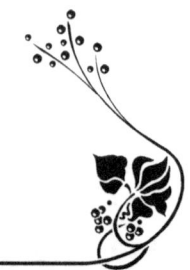

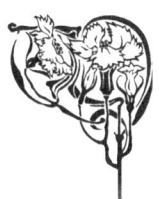

Apricot and Bee Honey
Face Mask
Normal or Dry Skin

What you need

1 apricot
1 teaspoon of sour cream
1 teaspoon of bee honey
20 grams of dry chamomile flowers

What to do

As we know, dry skin will always age faster than the other types. If this is your case, then take one fresh apricot and put it in a blender for ten to fifteen seconds. On the other hand, if you have a normal skin complexion, use a fruit squeezer to extract the apricot juice instead. In either case, mix well your apricot ingredient with sour cream first, and then add the honey.

Using a cotton puff, gently cover the entire face with an even layer of your just-made cream. Relax for ten to fifteen minutes, then wash off the mask with warm water. Dry with a clean paper towel and immediately apply a warm chamomile extract compress for ten minutes. When done, do not wash your face. Let it dry.

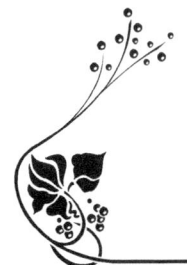

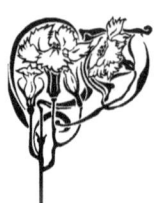

Banana - Musa Paradisiaca

Health and Beauty Benefits

Use this recipe in order to regain the shine and elasticity of your skin.

Highly concentrated in iron and potassium, bananas can stimulate the production of hemoglobin in the blood, thus working as anti-aging products. For this reason, for thousands of years, some cultures have regarded bananas as some of nature's secret fruits for perpetual youth.

Bananas have a powerful ability to increase the body's resistance to diseases. Also, eating bananas daily is beneficial to controlling high blood pressure.

Natural Properties

Vitamins: A, B1, B2, C and E
Minerals: Iron, Magnesium, Phosphorus, Potassium and Zinc.

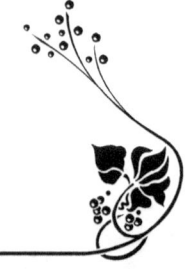

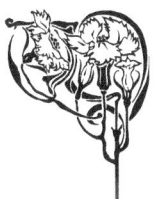

Banana and Bee Honey
Face Mask *Dry Skin Complexion*

What you need

> 1 ripe banana
> 1 teaspoon of bee honey

What to do

Take one well ripe banana and mush it in a blender at slow speed for thirty seconds. Add the honey to this thick, milky paste and then blend together for thirty more seconds.

Cleanse your skin well with either one of the cleansers suggested in this book (apple or linden), or with warm water and unscented soap. With a cotton ball well dipped into your fresh banana-honey cream, gently, cover your entire face with an even layer. Relax for ten to fifteen minutes. Wash the mask off with warm chamomile infusion and then apply a warm chamomile compress for ten more minutes. When done, do not wipe. Let it all soak into the skin.

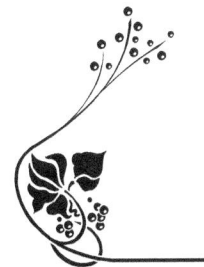

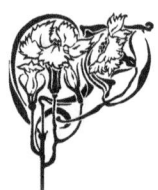

Banana - Musa Paradisiaca

Health and Beauty Benefits

Feeds and soothes your face skin since both banana oil and orange juice contain excellent nutrients. Read more about the properties of bananas on the previous page.

Natural Properties

Rich in fiber content and carbohydrates, and containing high levels of natural sugars, bananas are a good source of natural energy.

Vitamins: A, B, and C
Minerals: Iron, Magnesium, Phosphorus, Potassium
and Zinc.

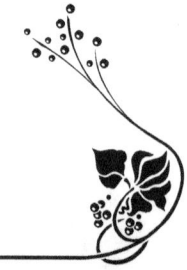

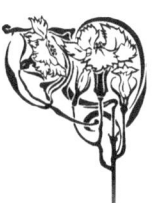

Masca de Banane with Sour Cream and Orange Juice *Oily Skin Complexion*

What you need

    1 banana
    1 teaspoon of sour cream
    1 teaspoon of orange juice

What to do

Blend together all ingredients in a blender at slow speed for fifteen seconds. With a cotton ball well dipped into your freshly made cream, cover gently your entire face with an even layer.

Relax for ten to fifteen minutes.

Wash off with warm water and let dry (do not wipe). Feel how supple your skin is now.

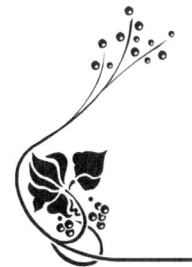

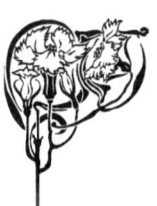

Honey - Mel

Health and Beauty Benefits

Bee honey has been used as a beauty ingredient for many thousands of years going as far back as the ancient Egypt and the Roman Empire.

It has softening and moisturizing characteristics, thus permitting the skin to rehydrate itself. It has a very pleasant, natural perfume. However, be warned that, if you are allergic to bee pollen, you may also be allergic to bee honey.

Natural Properties

Honey contains pretty much all the vitamins, especially A, B1, B2, B6, C, E and H. It is also very rich in enzymes and amino acids. Among others, we can find in its composition sugar, wax and acids such as citric, malic formic and lactic.

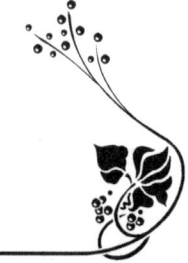

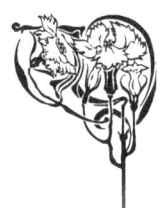

Bee Honey and Sunflower Oil Face Mask

Dry Skin Complexion

What you need

> 1 tablespoon of bee honey
> 1 tablespoon of natural sunflower oil
> 1 egg yolk

What to do

Take one fresh egg and carefully separate the yolk in a glass bowl. With a stir stick, mix the egg yolk well while you pour in a little bit of sunflower oil at the time. When all the oil has been used up, keep stirring while adding the honey this time. Continue until all the honey has been absorbed.

Wash your face well with warm water and unscented soap or one of my cleansers (linden or apple). Then, and while your skin is still moist, apply the mask with a cotton ball. Relax for ten to fifteen minutes and then wash off with warm water followed by a massage with infusion of chamomile.

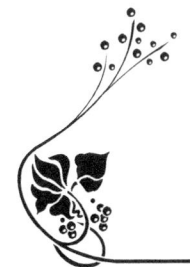

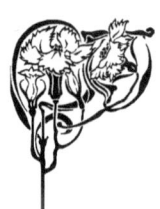

Cantaloupe - Cucumis Melo

Health and Beauty Benefits

Use for dry skin complexions. Cantaloupe and watermelon are low-calory, nutrition-packed fruits, both sitting at the very top of the health benefits charts. They are considered to be the best skin tissue regenerators.

Cantaloupe contains "adenosine", a natural compound highly beneficial to blood because it maintains it thin.

Cantaloupe juice contains nearly 100% of the fruit's nutritional values.

Natural Properties

Cantaloupe has high contents of vitamins A, B, B6, P and is a good source of fiber and acids: niacin, folic and pantothenic; also contains thiamine and carotenes.

Minerals: Calcium, Copper, Iron, Magnesium, Manganese, Phosphorus, Potassium, Zinc.

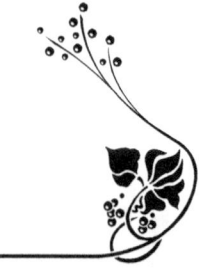

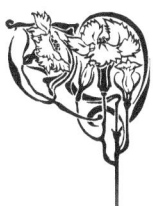

Cantaloupe and Milk Face Mask
Dry Skin Complexion

What you need

> 1 half of a fresh cantaloupe
> 1 tablespoon of 3.25% milk

What to do

Cut one half of a cantaloupe in pieces and using a fruit juicer, collect the juice. Mix about 30 grams of cantaloupe juice with the milk. For a later use you can freeze the remaining cantaloupe juice but do not yet mixed with milk.

Use this cream to massage your face gently with a cosmetic pad, nightly before bed time. Always remove with warm water and then massage with a cosmetic sponge soaked in a warm linden infusion. Do not wipe; let the linden be absorbed by your skin while you sleep.

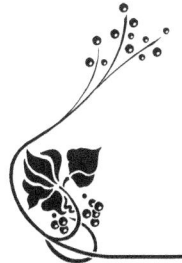

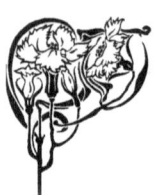

Chamomile - Matricaria Chamomilla

Health and Beauty Benefits

Use this heavenly healthy infusion as a skin cleanser, massaging ingredient and face mask remover.

This is what I consider to be the most important of all old health and beauty secrets revealed to me by my grand mother who is an expert in extracting fragrances and vitamins from plants and fruits. And, believe me, she has no fancy lab. She does it all on her old kitchen stove. In fact, she's been doing it for over 70 years now!

Natural Properties

Chamomile has strong anti-inflammatory properties; it is considered bactericidal, anti-itching, soothing, antiseptic, purifying, refreshing and hypoallergenic, thus being able to neutralize, pretty much, all skin irritants!!! It is aromatic. It is an excellent non-comedogenic natural product so it can be beneficial in use after shaving; very efficient in eye treatment preparations for dry and super sensitive skin. It can be used for burns. Chamomile herb has a great contribution to the delay and removal of wrinkles.

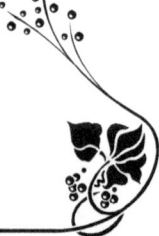

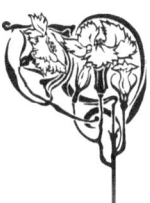

Chamomile Infusion and Extract as Cleanser

Oily Skin Complexion

What you need

> 20 grams of dry chamomile flowers
> 200 grams of distilled water

What to do

Ladies, please pay particular attention to this short recipe, as you'll be also needing chamomile extract or infusion for just about every other recipe in this book.

In a glass bowl, pour 50 grams of cold water on top of the dry chamomile flowers and cover for five minutes. Then pour 200 grams of boiling hot water on top and let simmer for twenty minutes. Filter through a paper filter in a clean cup.

Using cotton pads as compresses well soaked in this infusion, cover your face for twenty minutes, nightly before bed time. Also, properly prepared, chamomile can be used to loose weight. See beauty tips at end of the book.

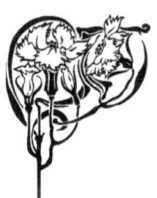

Cherry - Prunus Cerasus

Health and Beauty Benefits

Anti-wrinkle; use when very tired and whenever you feel that your face's skin "needs a holiday".

When properly eaten with other foods, cherries are very effective in weight loss.

Natural Properties

Viewed for generations as a "super fruit" while being an extremely powerful anti-oxidant, cherry is considered to have the highest capability to fight disease including diabetes and some cancers.

Vitamins: A, B, and C
Minerals: Chlorine, Cobalt, Copper, Magnesium, Manganese, Phosphorus, Potassium, Sulfur, Zinc. Also contains Melatonin. (Wow!)

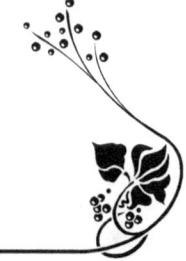

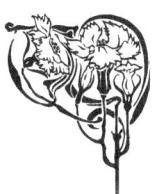

Cherry Face Mask

Normal Skin Complexion

What you need

     one fist full of fresh red cherries

Warning! DO NOT USE CHERRIES IF YOU ARE ALLERGIC TO THEM!

What to do

Because cherries have such a high content of vitamins and minerals, there's no need to mix or blend them with any other fruits or natural juices.

For a very tired skin complexion, mush 6 to 10 seedless cherries and apply them to your face for fifteen minutes.

Wash off with cold chamomile or linden infusion.

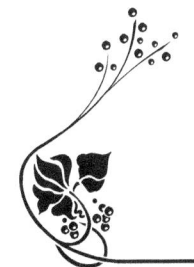

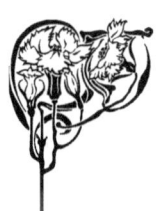

Egg Yolk - Vitellus

Health and Beauty Benefits

Egg yolk's content of vitamin A and lecithin sterols makes it a prime candidate for dry, sensitive skin care. By allowing the skin to build up a supply of water, the egg yolk has smoothing and nutrient qualities; it, thus, provides a temporary tightening effect of the skin.

Natural Properties

Egg yolk is one of the few foods that contain high concentrations of natural vitamin D.

Vitamins: B, B6, D and E
Very Rich in: Proteins, Oils, Calcium Phosphates, Sodium and Magnesium.

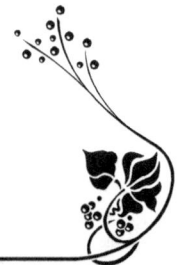

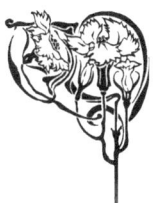

Egg Yolk and Olive Oil Face Mask
Dry Skin Complexion

What you need

> 1 egg yolk
> 1 tablespoon of olive oil
> 1 teaspoon of bee honey
> 1 capsule of vitamin A

What to do

Mix well one egg yolk with the olive oil, then add the honey and the content of one capsule of vitamin A (yes, the same vitamine A that you buy regularly from your local drug store). Continue to mix all the ingredients until you obtain a creamy paste.

Use this cream to cover your face with an even film coat. Make sure to avoid application around the eyes. Wait for fifteen minutes and then remove with warm water. Do not wipe; let dry.

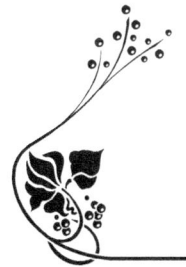

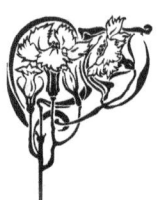

Grapefruit - Citrus Paradisi

Health and Beauty Benefits

Grapefruit is beneficial for oily skin types. It has antiseptic antiseptic properties and a high content of vitamin C. In high concentrations it is too caustic to use on the face. It could produce reactions in sensitive skin people.

Grapefruit juice is a natural activator for the nutrition functions of skin's cells. Having toning and astringent effects, grapefruit enhances skin's vitality and helps it regain its elasticity and shine. For these reasons I recommend that you use this recipe several times a week.

Natural Properties

Vitamins: B, B2, and C
Minerals: Calcium, Chlorophyll, Iron, Magnesium, Phosphorus, Potassium and enzymes.

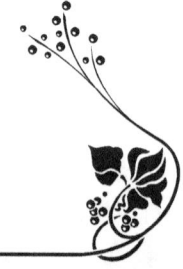

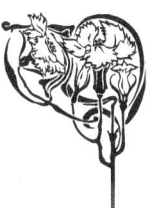

Grapefruit Face Mask

Oily Skin Complexion

What you need

1 teaspoon of grapefruit
1 teaspoon of sour cream
1 egg white
500 grams of mineral water

What to do

Blend well an egg white until it turns in the usual white, foamy cream we all know so well from our weekly routine of baking and cooking.

Now, add to it the sour cream and grapefruit juice and blend for thirty more seconds.

Apply this paste to your face and wait fifteen minutes before you remove it with mineral water.

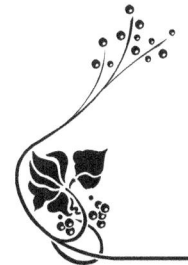

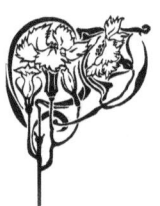

Grape - Vitis Vinifera

Health and Beauty Benefits

Grapes combat wrinkles and are well known for their natural property to increase the elasticity of face muscles and thus, skin's shine.

Use white grapes for normal skin, and red grapes only for oily skin complexions (could stain).

Most of the health benefits of the grapes are concentrated in their skin, not the pulp. They are excellent sources of antioxidants and are also very rich in flavonoids.

Natural Properties

Vitamins: A, B, and C
Minerals: Calcium, Iron, Magnesium, Phosphorus
Potassium and Selenium.

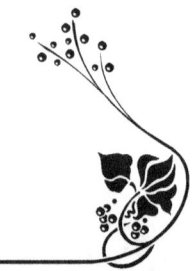

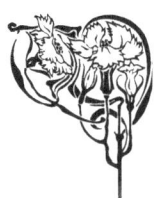

Grapes and Corn Powder as Skin Revitalizers *Normal Skin Complexion*

What you need

> 1 teaspoon of natural white grape juice
> 1 tablespoon of lemon juice
> 1 or 2 table spoons of corn powder
> 1 egg white

What to do

Mix well and slowly ALL the ingredients until you obtain an homogeneous cream, then apply it evenly to your well cleaned skin.

Wait for fifteen minutes.

Remove only with a cosmetic sponge soaked in a fresh, warm infusion of chamomile.

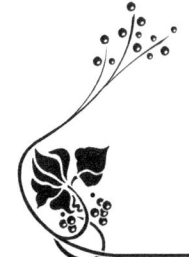

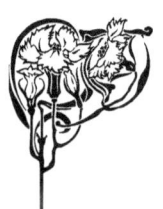

Linden - Tilia Spp.

Health and Beauty Benefits

Linden is an excellent antiseptic, skin cleansing solution, soothing sedative and blood circulation stimulant. In a shell, this is the ONLY other natural infusion and cleanser that can, possibly, top the benefits of chamomile.

If the instructions on preparing the linden infusion sound very much like making tea or coffee, believe me - it isn't! It's a whole different chemical process. Don't try to cheat and rush it by using a coffee maker 'cause that won't do! This slow process represents the secret key, the "magic" and powers of this cleanser. Believe me, I didn't invent this process; I learned them from very, old people, who themselves were taught by other very, very old people, who themselves...

Natural Properties

Vitamins: B, B2, and C
Minerals: Calcium, Chlorophyll, Iron, Magnesium, Phosphorus, Potassium and enzymes.

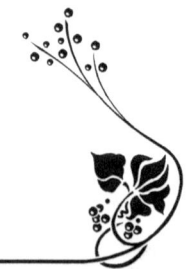

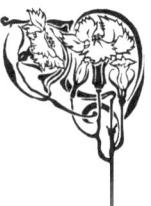

Linden Infusion as Cleanser

Oily Skin Complexion

What you need

>250 grams of water
>20 grams of linden leaves

What to do

Bring 150 grams of water to a full boil. Take 10 grams of linden leaves and add them to your water. Do not stir or sink the leaves into the water. Just cover with a glass top and let sit for about fifteen minutes after which filter it through a paper filter in a clean cup. This will slowly extract from leaves almost 100% of all their natural ingredients. Let this "tea" cool off slowly until it reaches room temperature or until you are comfortable to use it.

When ready, apply it to your entire face and over your closed eyes, in form of compress. Right away, you will notice a cool, clean, soft and moist feel of your skin. Let it dry for twenty minutes, then wash face with warm water. The end benefits of linden infusion are spectacular, mainly when the eyes are very tired. While bed time use will do, I recommend that you do this routine first thing in the morning.

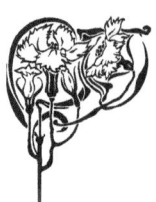

Linden - Tilia Spp.

Health and Beauty Benefits

As I mentioned on the previous page, linden is an excellent antiseptic, a skin cleansing solution, a soothing sedative and an excellent blood circulation stimulant.

Yet, linden offers lots more health and beauty benefits, one of which is that it can also be used it as a "bath salt" for relaxation of muscle tension and common colds.

Please notice that in the preparation of both linden extract and linden infusion, I am not using the linden "flowers". This is very important to remember because most natural health applications of the linden are associated with its flowers. However, for skin maintenance, we need *linden leaves*.

Natural Properties

Vitamins: B, B2, and C
Minerals: Calcium, Chlorophyll, Iron, Magnesium, Phosphorus, Potassium and enzymes.

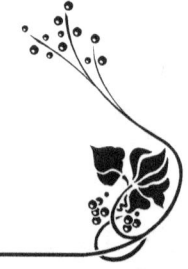

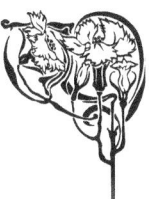

Linden Extract - a Wrinkle Fighter

Normal Skin Complexion

What you need

> 250 grams of water
> 20 grams of linden leaves

What to do

In order to use linden as a wrinkle fighter, you will want to use it nightly before you go to bed:

In 250 grams of boiled water soak 10 grams of linden leaves for about five minutes. Strain the used leaves and let this solution to cool to room temperature or until comfortably warm. Massage your face well with a cotton pad soaked in this solution. Needless to say, emphasize on the portions of your face where the wrinkles are prominent. Do not wipe. Let dry and in the morning wash your face with warm water.

Use linden daily in form of a compress. Also, use it often as a face mask remover.

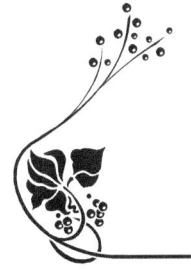

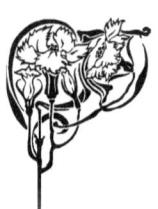

Wild Strawberry - Fraga

Health and Beauty Benefits

From the very beginning I advise you to be cautious since wild strawberries could create reactions in some people who are also known to be allergic to strawberries.

Wild strawberries, or "fragi", are a bit more difficult to obtain since they mostly grow in the remote areas height of mountains. For those of you who are not familiar with them, I can tell you that they look like very small strawberries (about 1/4" to 3/8"), are incredibly sweet and have an indescribably strong and pleasant fragrance and flavor. In Latin, "fragaria" means "fragrance"...

Equally, wild strawberries seem to have magic powers in fighting wrinkles and relaxing the facial muscles.

Natural Properties

Vitamins: B, C, and E.
Minerals: Calcium, Iodine, Iron, Magnesium,
                Potassium, Sodium and Sulfur.

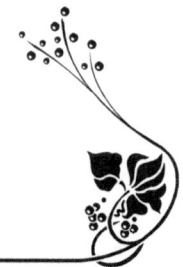

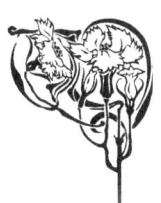

Masca de Fragi (Wild Strawberries Face Mask)
Oily Skin Complexion

What you need

> 2 teaspoons of wild strawberries
> 1 teaspoon of olive oil
> 1 teaspoon of sour cream

What to do

To start with, you need 20 to 30 grams of wild strawberries which, before using, you have to make sure that they've been washed very well.

Mush them with a fork on a plate and then mix them well with the olive oil. Add the sour cream.

Clean your face well. Apply this mask throughout your face. Wait ten to fifteen minutes and then wash off with warm water.

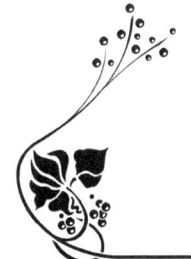

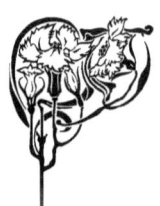

Oranges - Citrus Aurantium

Health and Beauty Benefits

This is an antispasmodic combination with softening and sedative properties benefiting delicate skins.

This particular combination of fruits represents a multitude of vitamins and natural products, too many to enumerate. Please see the other recipes included in this collection for references.

Natural Properties

Oranges contain beta-carotene and bioflavonoids, calcium, folic acid and vitamins and minerals...

Vitamins: A, B1, B6 and C,
Minerals: Iron, Magnesium and Potassium.

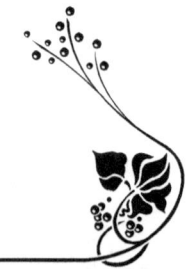

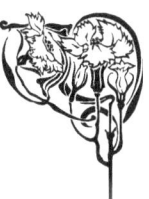

Oranges and Apples as Skin Softeners

Oily Skin Complexion

What you need

> 1 orange
> 1 apple
> 15 grams of bee honey

What to do

Take one fresh orange and one peeled, coreless apple and mush them in a fruit juicer until they turn into juice. Add to this juice 15 grams of pure bee honey and blend together for thirty seconds. Pour the mixture in a glass bowl and let settle for ten minutes. Meanwhile, cleanse your skin well with warm water and unscented soap.

With a cotton puff well soaked into your freshly made cream, gently cover all your face with an even layer.

Relax for ten to fifteen minutes. Wash the mask off with a warm, sugarless infusion of chamomile. Wipe gently with a paper towel.

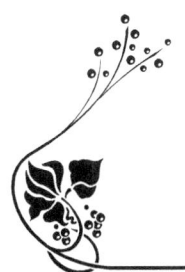

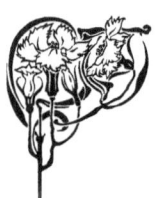

Peach - Prunus Persica

Health and Beauty Benefits

Peaches are very beneficial for dry skin because they have powerful toning properties which help tighten and strengthen the elasticity of skin tissues. This makes them very effective in wrinkle preventive uses. Overall, the use of peach fruit will bring back the elasticity and shine of your skin.

Peach is mainly used when your face is very tired and the wrinkles tend to appear. It also protects your skin against external agents such as wind, dryness, cold air and sun.

Peaches can also be used in aromatherapy and can be often found as natural ingredient in many bath soaps and deodorants.

Natural Properties

Vitamins: A, B, C and E
Minerals: Phosphorus, Potassium and Magnesium and Fatty acids.

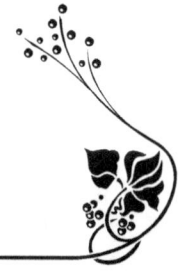

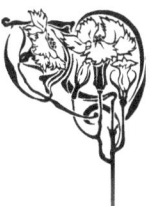

Peach Face Mask

Dry Skin Complexion

What you need

    1 well ripe peach
    1 teaspoon of sour cream
    1 capsule of vitamin A

What to do

Mush well one seedless peach in your blender for about fifteen seconds. Add the sour cream and the content of one capsule of vitamin A and mix for another fifteen seconds.

Apply the paste you obtain to your face and wait for fifteen minutes after which time you will remove it with warm water.

Wipe with a paper towel then massage your face with a cotton pad and chamomile infusion.

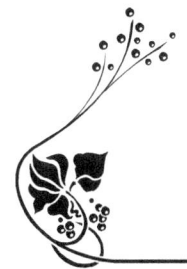

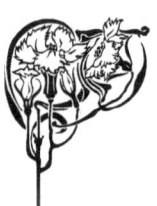

Pineapple - Ananas

Health and Beauty Benefits

Pineapple is very rich in amino acids and enzymes and has excellent exfoliating properties. It is also an excellent relaxant, skin nutrient and rehydrant.

Pineapple is can be used with amazing results in weight loss (see the beauty tips at the end of the book). However, when used for skin care purposes, be warn as for some people pineapple can be an irritant.

Natural Properties

Pineapple has natural anti-inflammatory properties, thus accelerating healing. It can be used effectively in the treatment of bruises.

Vitamins: A, B, and C
Minerals: Calcium, Potassium, Iodine, Iron, Magnesium, Phosphorus.

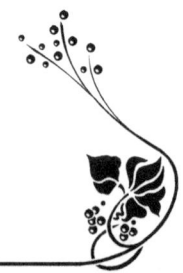

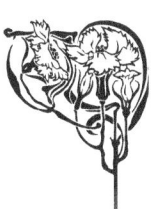

Pineapple Cleanser

Dry Skin Complexion

What you need

1 half of a fresh pineapple

What to do

This routine is as beneficial to your skin as it is simple!

Cut the pineapple in very thin slices, as you would cut a cucumber.

Apply these slices to your pre-cleaned face for twenty minutes. Relax.

When done, wash your face off with warm linden infusion.

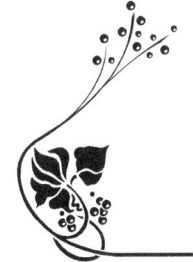

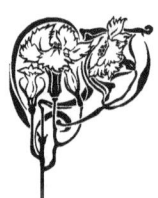

Strawberry - Fragaria Vesca

Health and Beauty Benefits

Strawberries sooth the skin and can also serve as an excellent remedy for treating sunburn areas.

Strawberries contain pectin, malic and citric acids, sugar and water. But, they are also one of the foods most commonly associated with allergic reactions.

Note: If you (think) you are allergic to strawberries, STAY AWAY from this recipe!

Natural Properties

Vitamins: B2, B5, B6, C and K.
Minerals: Calcium, Chlorophyll, Copper, Iodine, Magnesium, Manganese, Potassium and Omega 3 fatty acids (!!!)

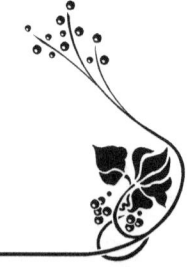

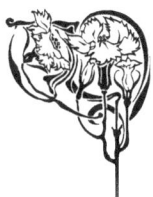

Strawberries & Sour Cream face Mask
Dry Skin Complexion

What you need

> 3 strawberries
> 1 tablespoon of sour cream
> 1 capsule of vitamin E

What to do

Take three strawberries and blend them at high speed for fifteen seconds. Add to them one tablespoon of sour cream and the content of a capsule of vitamin E. (Sour cream has high nutritive and therapeutic properties because it's composition is based on enzymes and bacterial cultures).

Blend again for thirty seconds. You will obtain a pink, (delicious too) milky cream which is a very healthy skin nutrient.

Apply this mask with a cotton puff, in an even layer, to your well pre-cleaned face. Relax for fifteen minutes, then remove the mask with warm chamomile infusion.

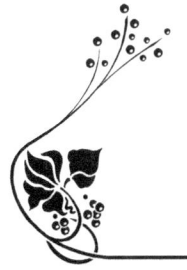

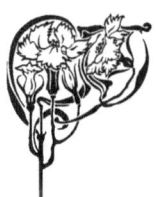

Vinegar - Armeniaca Vulgaris

Health and Beauty Benefits

This recipe can be used for healthy results with all types of skin and hair.

Dandruff is the product of an unhealthy scalp skin. So, my advise is that, once you start this routine, you should repeat it every other day for one week. Soon, you will notice the obvious, if not total disappearance of the unwanted flakes. Continuing this process periodically, once to twice a week, you will also prevent dandruff from coming back. But remember, do not over do it and, most importantly, **do not get any in your eyes!**

Natural Properties

Vinegar has been around for so long that no one really knows when, or where, it has first originated. For centuries, practically, every culture has been using vinegar as both a natural medication and a beauty ingredient. Vinegar is very rich in vitamins and minerals, in special Potassium. One of its most notable properties is that it has the power to normalize the body's acid levels (pH).

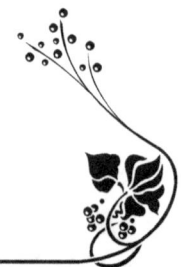

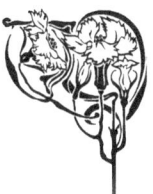

Vinegar as Dandruff Remover

All Skin and Hair Types

What you need

1.5 litre of warm water
35 grams of organic, white vinegar

What to do

In 1.5 litres of warm water pour 35 grams of pure white vinegar (5% acetic acid by vol.). Stir well, don't shake. First, wash your hair with warm water and plain, unscented soap. Use your finger tips to massage deeply the skin on your head. Rinse and wash a second time repeating the very same process. Rinse with water for the second time.

When all the soap is gone, rinse again, this time with this vinegar cleanser. It's best to ask someone to pour it slowly over your head while you make sure, very diligently, that you are not missing any parts of your hair. Use entire mixture. When done, cover your hair in a soft, warm towel and wait for about five minutes. Uncover and let dry while you untangle it with your hands. Once dried, brush it with a very clean and soft brush.

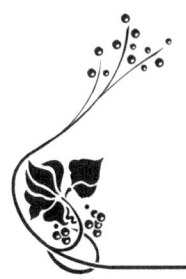

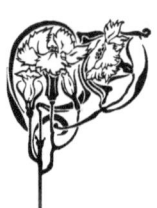

Beauty Tips

Did you know that...

Sour cream has high nutritive and therapeutic properties? This is because sour cream is based on enzymes and bacterial cultures.

Plain yogurt is an excellent remedy for sunburns; it is very rich in proteins, glucides and carbohydrates

You can avoid wrinkles by cleaning your face daily with pure apple juice for about five minutes.

You can loose weight by...

Eating pineapple daily, in the morning, on a empty stomach. Wait about two hours before you have your regular breakfast.

Drinking 300 grams of chamomile tea every morning, 15 to 20 minutes before breakfast (give this a couple of weeks before you will notice the difference on the scale).

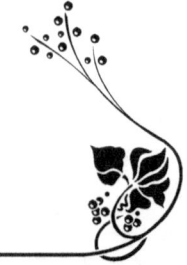

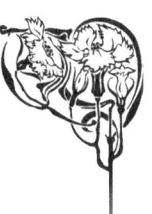

Glossary of Basic Terms

Antioxidant: (property): helps slow the aging process

Antiseptic: sterilizer, disinfectant, hygienic

Astringent: reduces the oil content on skin's surface

Exfoliate: discards the dead layers of skin

Hypoallergenic: does not produce allergic reactions

Non-comedogenic: won't plug skin's pores

Rehydrate: helps the skin to regain its moisture

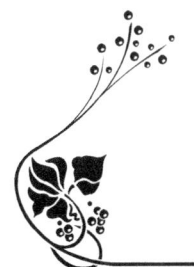

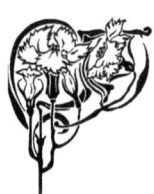

Your Beauty Notes

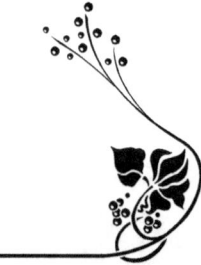

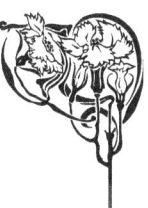

Your Beauty Notes

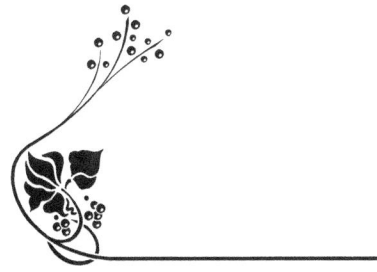

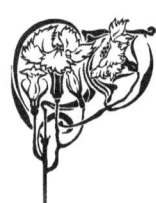

Stephanie's
Home Beauty Salon

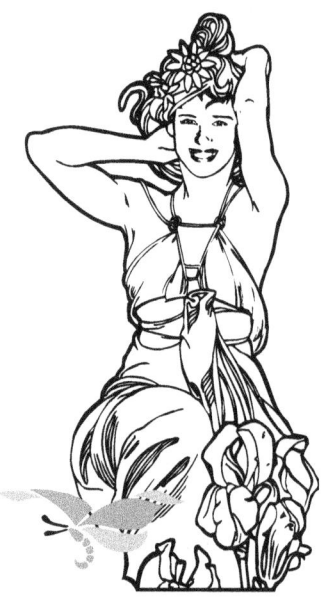

Stay Beautiful!

- Stephanie

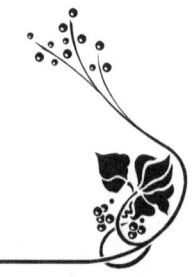

www.ingramcontent.com/pod-product-compliance
Lightning Source LLC
Chambersburg PA
CBHW060649290526
45793CB00001B/461